NATUROPATHIC MEDICINE PRINCIPLE

Complete Guide To Understanding Its Foundations, Diagnosis Principles, Treatment Modalities, Common Condition Approaches, And Integration With Conventional Medicine

WILFREDO CARSON

pg. 1

INTRODUCTION

Naturopathic Medicine is a holistic approach to healthcare that stresses the body's innate ability to repair itself naturally.

This type of medicine combines a range of traditional therapeutic traditions, modern scientific understanding, and personalized patient care. Naturopathic medicine's principles guide practitioners in addressing the underlying causes of illness and improving general health. Naturopathy stands apart from traditional medicine due to its holistic approach, which has earned it respect as an alternative or complementary healthcare method.

Overview of Naturopathic Medicine.

Naturopathic medicine comprises a wide range of therapeutic techniques that emphasize the body's inherent healing processes. This includes, but is not limited to, herbal medicine, diet, hydrotherapy, physical manipulation, and lifestyle advice. Practitioners strive to develop a personalized therapy plan for each patient, taking into account their unique physiological, psychological, and environmental characteristics.

The holistic nature of naturopathy is obvious in its emphasis on treating the whole person rather than isolated symptoms, with the ultimate objective of restoring balance and encouraging long-term health. This introduction lays the groundwork for a more in-depth look at the historical roots and development of naturopathic medicine.

<u>Historical Background:</u>

Naturopathic medicine has its roots in ancient healing systems from diverse civilizations, such as Ayurveda, Traditional Chinese Medicine, and Native American Medicine.

The concept that the body has an inbuilt potential to repair itself is a common thread running through these various practices. However, the contemporary concept of naturopathy arose in the late nineteenth century, thanks to the efforts of early pioneers such as Benedict Lust and Sebastian Kneipp. Benedict Lust, a German immigrant, is known as the "father of naturopathy" since he coined the term and established the first naturopathic college in the United States in the early twentieth century. The following development of naturopathic ideas and philosophy reflects a blend of traditional wisdom and increasing scientific knowledge.

<u>Principles and philosophy:</u>

Naturopathic medicine is guided by six essential concepts that serve as the foundation of its philosophy. These principles serve as a foundation for diagnosis, treatment, and patient care, with an emphasis on a comprehensive and patient-centered approach.

1. The Healing Power of Nature: The first principle acknowledges the body's intrinsic ability to heal itself. Naturopathic practitioners believe that the body has a vital force or life energy that, when nurtured, may overcome illness and restore balance. This idea emphasizes the significance of recognizing and removing barriers to healing

while also assisting the body's natural processes.

2. Identify and Treat the Causes: Naturopathy seeks to address the underlying causes of sickness rather than simply relieving symptoms. Practitioners undertake detailed exams to discover underlying causes such as inadequate diet, environmental pollutants, and emotional stress. Naturopathic medicine aims to prevent health problems from recurring and improve long-term well-being by addressing the underlying causes.

3. First, Do No Harm (Primum Non-Nocere): This principle is consistent with the Hippocratic Oath, emphasizing the reduction of harm in the quest for healing. Naturopathic interventions highlight the use of non-invasive, low-risk remedies, emphasizing the

necessity of avoiding unnecessary side effects or problems. This dedication to the least harmful technique is consistent with the overarching goal of increasing overall patient safety.

4. Doctor as Teacher (Docere): Naturopathic practitioners serve as both doctors and educators. They provide patients with information and insight about their health, promoting active engagement in the healing process. Naturopathic doctors strive to provide clients with the skills they need to make informed decisions about their health by cultivating a collaborative partnership.

5. Treat the Whole Person: Naturopathic philosophy is founded on the concept that health and disease are influenced by a

complex interplay of physical, mental, emotional, and environmental variables.

Rather than focusing solely on symptoms or organs, naturopathic medicine takes into account their interdependence. This holistic approach provides a thorough insight into the individual, directing tailored treatment options.

6. Naturopathy emphasizes preventive care, to identify and address possible health issues before they become illnesses. This proactive approach entails teaching patients on good lifestyle choices, stress management techniques, and illness prevention tactics. Naturopathic medicine aims to reduce future health difficulties by increasing total well-being.

These concepts establish the conceptual foundation of naturopathic medicine and guide practitioners' approaches to patient care. The use of these concepts distinguishes naturopathy from traditional medical methods by emphasizing a patient-centered, preventive, and holistic approach to healthcare.

CHAPTER 1
FOUNDATIONS OF NATUROPATHIC MEDICINE

Naturopathic medicine is based on a set of fundamental principles that govern its approach to healing and well-being.

These ideas take a holistic approach, recognizing the interdependence of the body, mind, and spirit. One of the basic pillars is the concept of vital force, which is essential in the healing process. Furthermore, a holistic approach is stressed, treating the entire person rather than just the symptoms. Furthermore, naturopathic medicine lays a strong focus on nature's healing potential, regarding it as a valuable source of medicine and incorporating a variety of natural remedies into its practice.

<u>The Vital Force</u>

The concept of vital force is central to the naturopathic medical philosophy.

Based on vitalism, this notion asserts the existence of a life force or energy that animates living entities and promotes health. Vitalism contends that the body possesses an intrinsic intelligence that orchestrates the healing process.

Naturopathic practitioners think that sustaining and increasing this vital force can help restore balance and well-being. Understanding vitalism is acknowledging the body's natural potential to heal itself when given the correct conditions. This viewpoint is consistent with the holistic character of naturopathy, which goes beyond treating symptoms to address underlying imbalances that may impair the vital force.

Naturopathic medicine focuses on the vital force to boost the body's self-healing mechanisms and restore maximum health.

The vital force plays a varied role in healing. Symptoms, according to Naturopathic practitioners, are indications of an underlying imbalance in vital energy, rather than discrete ailments. Rather than simply suppressing symptoms, the emphasis is on identifying and treating the underlying causes.

This approach is consistent with the notion of treating the complete person, understanding that physical problems are frequently caused by psychological, emotional, or environmental causes.

Naturopathic treatment seeks to promote long-term healing by restoring vital force balance. This perspective distinguishes naturopathy from conventional medicine by emphasizing the body's natural ability to maintain and restore health.

Holistic Approach

Naturopathic medicine takes a holistic approach, acknowledging the complex interplay of an individual's body, mind, and spirit. The holistic perspective recognizes that health and well-being are influenced by elements other than the physical body. Treating the full person requires taking into account the interconnectivity of physiological, psychological, and spiritual elements. Naturopathic practitioners consider an individual's lifestyle, mental well-being, social surroundings, and spiritual beliefs, recognizing that all of these aspects influence total health.

The mind-body link is important to naturopathic medicine's holistic approach.

The complex interaction between mental and physical health is acknowledged and addressed during the treatment process. Stress, emotions, and mental attitudes are viewed as potential causes of illness or elements that can impede the healing process. Counseling, mindfulness, and stress reduction techniques are common practices used in naturopathic interventions to promote mental and emotional well-being.

Naturopathic medicine, by addressing the mind-body connection, seeks to promote not just physical health but also emotional and mental well-being, fostering a comprehensive approach to healing.

<u>The Healing Power of Nature</u>

Nature is seen as a potent source of medicine in naturopathic philosophy. This principle is based on the belief that the body has the innate ability to repair itself when given the correct conditions. Nature offers a wide variety of healing treatments, including herbal medicine, diet, hydrotherapy, and physical activity. Naturopathic practitioners use natural remedies to promote the body's internal healing capabilities.

Nature as a source of medicine includes the use of botanical treatments made from plants that have therapeutic characteristics. Herbal medicine, a cornerstone of naturopathic therapy, is the use of plant-based compounds to treat a variety of health issues.

These natural molecules are thought to act in tandem with the body, offering therapeutic benefits while avoiding the adverse effects commonly associated with pharmaceutical medications. Furthermore, naturopathic nutrition emphasizes the necessity of a healthy and balanced diet, knowing that food is more than just a source of nourishment; it is also a form of medicine that can influence health outcomes.

Naturopathic therapies are based on nature's healing potential and include techniques such as hydrotherapy, which uses water in various forms such as baths, compresses, and wraps to induce recovery. Physical activity, another cornerstone of natural therapy, is emphasized as an essential component of preserving health. These therapies are intended to assist the body's natural processes, increase vitality, and restore equilibrium. Naturopathic medicine strives to enhance the environment for the vital force to function optimally, allowing for a holistic and sustainable approach to health and wellness.

CHAPTER 2
PRINCIPLES OF NATUROPATHIC DIAGNOSIS

Patient-Centered Evaluation: Naturopathic medicine takes a comprehensive approach to patient care, and patient-centered evaluation is central to its diagnostic principles. This entails diving into the individual's whole health history, realizing that health is defined by more than just the absence of sickness, but also by the balance and harmony that exists across the entire person. Naturopathic practitioners take the time to acquire extensive information about their patients' previous and present health issues, lifestyle choices, dietary habits, stress levels, and environmental exposures. This deep grasp of the patient's health journey enables naturopathic physicians to recognize the interconnectivity of numerous aspects affecting their well-being. Naturopathic practitioners lay the groundwork for personalized and effective treatment options by focusing the diagnostic process on the patient.

Physical examinations, in addition to a full health history, are critical components of naturopathic medicine's patient-centered assessment. Unlike conventional medicine, which may focus on specific symptoms or organ systems, naturopathic physical examinations seek to assess the individual's overall vitality and balance.

Palpation, observation, and other noninvasive methods are used to evaluate the body's structural integrity, vital signs, and physiological functioning.

 Naturopathic practitioners obtain a more sophisticated view of their patient's health status by integrating these physical examinations with information gathered from the health history. This tailored and detailed approach enables the detection of small imbalances and early symptoms of malfunction, directing the development of focused and comprehensive treatment strategies.

Integrative diagnostic: Naturopathic medicine uses the integrative diagnostic theory to bridge the gap between conventional and alternative healthcare techniques. This approach recognizes the benefits of both conventional and naturopathic methods and advocates their combined use to gain a more complete picture of the patient's health. Integrative diagnosis entails a partnership between naturopathic physicians and other healthcare experts, who recognize that multiple medical modalities can provide unique insights and contribute to a more comprehensive diagnosis.

Naturopathic practitioners may use conventional diagnostic methods including laboratory tests, imaging scans, and other medical assessments in integrated diagnosis. These tools provide objective data that can be used to identify specific illness signs. Naturopathic medicine, on the other hand, goes beyond these traditional methods by incorporating a wider range of diagnostic approaches. Naturopathic diagnostic tools include assessing nutritional status, evaluating lifestyle factors, and taking emotional well-being into account. By combining these many diagnostic methods, naturopathic practitioners acquire a more detailed picture of the underlying causes of a patient's health.

Identifying the Root Cause: At the foundation of naturopathic diagnosis is a commitment to identifying and resolving the source of health problems. Instead of simply treating symptoms, naturopathic practitioners aim to identify the root causes of an individual's health problems. This approach is consistent with the naturopathic belief that symptoms are expressions of the body's desire to restore balance and should be regarded as useful indicators rather than nuisances.

Addressing underlying disorders in naturopathic medicine entails delving into the complex web of elements that influence health, such as lifestyle, food, stressors, environmental exposures, and genetic predisposition. Naturopathic physicians conduct a thorough evaluation of the patient's medical history and use diagnostic instruments to detect physiological imbalances, dietary deficiencies, and other contributing variables. Understanding the core reason allows naturopathic practitioners to develop treatment regimens that not only relieve symptoms but also promote long-term health and prevent the recurrence of health problems.

Individualized Treatment Programs: Naturopathic medicine acknowledges the uniqueness of each individual, and this philosophy extends to the creation of individualized treatment programs. After identifying the fundamental cause through a patient-centered evaluation and integrative diagnosis, naturopathic practitioners develop individualized treatment solutions based on the patient's specific needs, preferences, and circumstances. This method differs from the one-size-fits-all strategy prevalent in conventional medicine.

Individualized treatment regimens in naturopathy include a variety of therapeutic techniques such as diet, botanical medicine, acupuncture, hydrotherapy, and lifestyle counseling. These treatments are chosen based on their potential to address the underlying problem and stimulate the body's natural healing mechanisms. Naturopathic doctors work with patients to set realistic and attainable health goals, stressing empowerment and active participation in the healing process. The customized nature of naturopathic treatment regimens allows for flexibility and adaptation over time, ensuring that the approach remains in sync with the dynamic character of an individual's health journey.

The concepts of naturopathic diagnosis emphasize a comprehensive and personalized approach to healthcare. Naturopathic medicine provides a complete and nuanced framework for promoting health and well-being by emphasizing patient-centered assessment, integrative diagnosis, determining the fundamental cause, and developing tailored treatment strategies. This theory not only addresses symptoms but also seeks to restore balance and harmony inside the body, promoting long-term vitality and resilience. Naturopathic diagnosis is a guiding principle in the practice of naturopathy, defining the practitioner's understanding of health and directing them to provide effective and customized care to their patients.

CHAPTER 3
NATUROPATHIC TREATMENT MODALITIES

Naturopathic medicine, as a holistic approach to healthcare, includes a wide range of therapeutic modalities aimed at enhancing the body's natural ability to heal itself.

Each modality is based on natural healing principles and aims to address the underlying causes of illness rather than simply treating symptoms. This comprehensive approach recognizes the interdependence of multiple biological systems and highlights the role of lifestyle variables in achieving optimal health.

Clinical Nutrition

Clinical nutrition, the foundation of naturopathic medicine, is critical in promoting the body's natural healing mechanisms.

The significance of nutrition in healing cannot be emphasized, as it offers the building blocks for cell repair and regeneration. Naturopathic practitioners stress the healing potential of foods and adjust dietary advice to individual needs. The addition of individualized therapeutic diets improves the efficacy of clinical nutrition by treating specific health concerns and optimizing nutritional balance. Naturopathic doctors work to empower people to make informed food choices that promote health and avoid disease by understanding the complex relationship between nutrition and general well-being.

<u>Herbal medicine.</u>

Herbal medicine, a traditional naturopathic practice, uses medicinal plants' curative powers to restore balance and vigor.

The medicinal plant overview covers a wide range of botanical species, each with its own set of therapeutic properties. Naturopathic practitioners skillfully create herbal treatments by combining several plant extracts to meet the diverse characteristics of health issues.

Herbal formulations are adjusted to individual needs, taking into account characteristics including constitution, symptoms, and underlying imbalances. This technique represents the holistic philosophy of naturopathic medicine, which uses the synergy of plant components to help the body's self-healing mechanisms.

<u>Homeopathy</u>

Homeopathy, founded on the idea of "like cures like," is a distinct and intricate branch of naturopathic medicine. The principles of homeopathic medicine call for the use of greatly diluted drugs that, in larger quantities, would elicit symptoms comparable to those being treated.

This paradoxical technique boosts the body's vital force, enabling self-healing. Constitutional prescribing in homeopathy is a sophisticated method that takes into account all of an individual's physical, mental, and emotional traits. Homeopathy, which individualizes treatment based on a person's unique constitution, resonates with naturopathy's holistic idea of restoring harmony on all levels.

Hydrotherapy

Hydrotherapy utilizes the healing potential of water, recognizing it as a versatile and powerful therapeutic agent. Hydrotherapeutic approaches involve the use of water in a variety of forms, temperatures, and applications. Water's capacity to regulate circulation, alleviate inflammation, and promote relaxation underpins its use in naturopathic medicine. Hydrotherapy methods range from simple hot and cold compresses to more complex procedures such as hydromassage and contrast baths. This method is consistent with naturopathic concepts, as it supports the body's natural functions, improves detoxification, and promotes general vitality.

<u>Physical Medicine</u>

Naturopathic physical medicine combines therapeutic exercise and manual therapies to treat musculoskeletal problems and improve healthy physical function. Therapeutic exercise is adapted to individual needs, with a focus on improving flexibility, strength, and overall mobility. Manual therapies include a variety of hands-on techniques such as massage, manipulation, and mobilization that aim to correct structural imbalances and promote tissue repair. This technique adheres to naturopathic principles by emphasizing the importance of physical well-being in overall health and using non-invasive therapies to restore balance.

Mind/Body Medicine

Naturopathic medicine recognizes the significant connection between the mind and body and incorporates mind-body therapies as an essential component of holistic therapy. Stress-reduction practices such as mindfulness meditation, yoga, and biofeedback are used to reduce the impact of stress on overall health. Naturopathy's concept of mental health goes beyond stress reduction to include more general characteristics of emotional well-being. Naturopathic practitioners understand the impact of mental and emotional states on physical health and work to help people achieve mental equilibrium as a core part of holistic therapy.

CHAPTER 4
NATUROPATHIC APPROACHES TO COMMON CONDITIONS

<u>Digestive Health</u>

Naturopathic medicine focuses a strong emphasis on digestive health, viewing the gastrointestinal system as a cornerstone of general wellness. The digestive system is vital for nutrient absorption, immunological function, and waste removal. Naturopathic methods for digestive issues use a holistic approach, aiming to address the underlying causes rather than simply treating symptoms. This frequently entails a thorough examination of food habits, lifestyle circumstances, and the individual's overall health. Typical naturopathic therapies include dietary adjustments, herbal supplements, and lifestyle changes focused on encouraging healthy digestion. Naturopathic practitioners seek to restore balance and harmony to the digestive system by focusing on the gut flora, acknowledging the delicate relationship between gut health and overall vitality.

The gut-brain connection

Naturopathic medicine acknowledges the complex relationship between the gut and the brain, stressing the bidirectional communication known as the gut-brain axis. This axis emphasizes the dynamic interaction between the central nervous system and the enteric neural system, which regulates gastrointestinal function. Imbalances in the gut microbiota can influence brain function and vice versa, affecting both mental health and digestive well-being. Naturopathic approaches to the gut-brain connection include therapies that support a healthy gut-bacteria balance, such as probiotics and prebiotics. In addition, stress management and mindfulness activities are used to address the psychosomatic component of digestive diseases. Understanding and managing the gut-brain connection is an essential component of naturopathic care for people with digestive health issues.

<u>Immunosystem Support</u>

Enhancing the Immune Response

Naturopathic medicine focuses on enhancing the body's natural ability to protect against infections and maintain normal immune function. Naturopathic practitioners seek to address the underlying causes of immune system abnormalities rather than simply treating symptoms.

Personalized dietary suggestions, nutritional supplementation, and lifestyle changes are all strategies for boosting the immune system. Naturopathic medicine emphasizes the value of a well-balanced diet high in vitamins, minerals, and antioxidants in maintaining immunological function. Herbal treatments, such as echinacea and astragalus, are commonly used to increase immunological strength. Naturopathic medicine seeks to enable the immune system to perform properly and sustain well-being by emphasizing holistic approaches that take into account the individual's total health.

<u>Preventive Measures</u>

In naturopathic medicine, prevention is regarded as a critical component of sustaining good health. Rather than waiting for sickness to strike, naturopathic practitioners collaborate with patients to develop proactive strategies to prevent immune system abnormalities.

This includes teaching patients on the benefits of a healthy lifestyle, such as good nutrition, frequent exercise, and stress management. Naturopathic preventive strategies also include the use of botanicals and supplements that have been shown to boost the immune system. Naturopathic medicine attempts to build a foundation that supports the body's natural defenses, minimizing the likelihood of sickness and promoting long-term health.

<u>Hormonal Balance.</u>

Naturopathic Solutions for Hormonal Issues

Hormonal balance is essential for overall health, as it influences a variety of physiological processes in the body. Naturopathic medicine acknowledges the interconnection of hormonal systems and seeks to treat hormonal abnormalities using natural and personalized methods. Naturopathic treatments for women's health frequently include dietary and lifestyle changes, as well as herbal therapies that promote hormonal balance at various phases of life. Similarly, naturopathic practitioners prioritize men's health by maximizing testosterone levels through lifestyle changes, dietary assistance, and tailored herbal therapies. Naturopathic medicine tailors interventions to address specific hormonal issues while taking into account each individual's unique biochemistry, to restore balance and promote general well-being.

<u>Women and Men's Health</u>

Naturopathic treatment acknowledges the distinct health needs of women and men, addressing gender-specific difficulties in a comprehensive and tailored manner. Naturopathic practitioners take the menstrual cycle, hormonal variations, and reproductive health into account when treating women. Nutritional supplements, botanical medicine, and lifestyle changes may be used to treat problems such as monthly irregularities, premenstrual syndrome (PMS), and menopausal symptoms. Naturopathic approaches to men's health focus on increasing testosterone levels, improving prostate health, and enhancing cardiovascular health. Naturopathic medicine tailors its interventions to meet the particular health needs of both men and women, creating balance and energy.

Chronic Pain Management

Naturopathic Treatments for Pain

Chronic pain is a serious burden for many people, affecting quality of life and frequently necessitating a thorough and integrative strategy. Naturopathic medicine treats chronic pain by taking into account the interdependence of physical, mental, and emotional health. Naturopathic pain management involves individualized treatment strategies that may include acupuncture, physical therapy, and mind-body treatments. Dietary therapies and nutritional support are also important because inflammation and vitamin imbalances can cause pain. Furthermore, herbal treatments having analgesic effects are frequently used to relieve pain naturally. Naturopathic medicine strives to promote overall well-being and quality of life for people suffering from chronic pain by addressing the underlying causes and using a comprehensive approach.

<u>Integrative Pain Treatments</u>

Naturopathic medicine promotes integrated pain therapies that blend conventional and alternative modalities to give comprehensive pain management. This may include including acupuncture, massage therapy, and chiropractic care into the treatment strategy. Mind-body methods such as meditation, yoga, and biofeedback are also used to treat the psychological and emotional elements of pain. Naturopathic practitioners collaborate with patients, taking a patient-centered approach to personalize interventions to their specific needs and preferences. Integrative pain therapies seek to promote balance and harmony within the body while also alleviating pain sensations. Naturopathic medicine offers a comprehensive and customized approach to chronic pain management by integrating evidence-based natural remedies with conventional treatments.

Naturopathic therapies for common diseases take a comprehensive and customized view of health and wellness. From digestive health to immune system support, hormone balance, and chronic pain management, naturopathic medicine aims to address the underlying causes of health imbalances and improve overall vitality.

The emphasis on preventive measures, understanding of the gut-brain connection, and individualized interventions for women's and men's health demonstrate the complete and patient-centered nature of naturopathic care. Naturopathic medicine combines evidence-based natural remedies with conventional approaches to empower people to take an active part in their health, promoting balance and well-being.

CHAPTER 5
INTEGRATING NATUROPATHY WITH CONVENTIONAL MEDICINE

Collaborative Healthcare: Naturopathy, as a holistic approach to healthcare, stresses the integration of many healing techniques, such as conventional medicine. Collaborative healthcare is a basic principle that emphasizes the value of naturopathic practitioners working alongside medical specialists.

The cooperation aims to provide patients with comprehensive and well-rounded therapy from both conventional and naturopathic viewpoints. This collaborative approach promotes open communication among practitioners from many professions, creating an atmosphere in which the strengths of each discipline can be harnessed for the benefit of patients. By recognizing the skills of medical experts and naturopathic practitioners, collaborative healthcare aims to bridge the gap between traditional and alternative medicine, thereby improving patient outcomes.

Interdisciplinary Care: The notion of interdisciplinary care is important to merging naturopathy and conventional medicine.

This entails the coordination and collaboration of healthcare providers from varied backgrounds to address all aspects of a patient's health. Naturopathic practitioners, who collaborate with medical experts, bring a distinct set of abilities and perspectives to the table. Interdisciplinary care recognizes that health is a complex notion, with different treatment methods making unique contributions.

Through collaborative efforts, practitioners hope to provide patients with a more thorough and tailored approach to their health. This approach recognizes that combining the benefits of naturopathy and conventional medicine can result in a more comprehensive and effective healthcare strategy.

Safety and efficacy:

Evidence-Based Naturopathy: Ensuring the safety and efficacy of naturopathic therapies is an essential component of competent healthcare practice. data-based naturopathy emphasizes the importance of using scientific data in naturopathic therapies. This strategy requires naturopathic practitioners to make recommendations based on well-established research, clinical studies, and empirical evidence.

By connecting naturopathic interventions with scientific rigor, practitioners can boost their field's legitimacy and foster confidence among patients and the broader medical community. Evidence-based naturopathy aims to eliminate myths about alternative therapies by establishing their efficacy via rigorous scientific research, ultimately helping to integrate naturopathy into mainstream healthcare.

Naturopathic Medicine Research: Research is critical to increasing awareness and acceptance of naturopathic medicine in the larger healthcare landscape. Conducting high-quality research in naturopathic medicine is critical for developing data to support the safety and efficacy of naturopathic therapies. This includes looking into the mechanisms of action, clinical outcomes, and potential negative effects of naturopathic treatments. Naturopathic practitioners give vital insights to the scientific community by conducting rigorous research, which promotes a more educated and evidence-based approach to patient care. Naturopathic medicine research also allows for collaboration with conventional medical experts, making it easier to integrate alternative medicines into mainstream healthcare procedures.

CONCLUSION

Naturopathic medicine's principles stress a whole-person, patient-centered approach to healthcare. Integrating naturopathy and conventional medicine is a step forward in providing individuals with comprehensive and well-rounded care. Collaborative healthcare, which involves naturopathic practitioners and medical specialists, guarantees that patients benefit from a wide spectrum of skills. Interdisciplinary care acknowledges the multidimensional character of health and promotes collaboration between various healthcare methods. Naturopathic medicine prioritizes safety and efficacy, with evidence-based methods and continuous research helping to build the field's legitimacy and acceptability within the medical world. As naturopathic concepts mature and align with scientific norms, the possibility for a harmonious integration of naturopathy and conventional medicine grows, eventually providing patients with a more holistic and customized approach to their well-being.